21 DAY TUMMY DIET JOURNAL
Weight Loss and Symptom Log

ISBN-13: 978-1505597936
ISBN-10: 1505597935

©2014 My Personal Journals
www.remarkableauthor.com/mpj

Free Gift for You

To get your free copy of

"How to Stay Motivated
and Lose Weight"

visit

www.staymotivatedclub.com/tummy

MEASURING YOUR SUCCESS

Weight Loss Chart

	Weight	Loss
Week 1		
Week 2		
Week 3		
Week 4		
Week 5		
Week 6		
Week 7		
Week 8		
Week 9		
Week 10		
Total Loss		

Body Measurements Chart

Measurement	Week 1	Week 3	Week 5	Week 7	Week 9	Inches Lost
Bust						
Chest						
Waist						
Hips						
Thigh						
Calves						
Upper arm						
Forearm						

BEFORE PICTURE

MY WEIGHT_____

WHAT I'M THINKING/HOW I FEEL: _____

_____
_____
_____
_____
_____
_____

WEEKLY MEAL PLANNER
Week of _____

	BREAKFAST	LUNCH	DINNER	SNACKS
MON				
TUE				
WED				
THU				
FRI				
SAT				
SUN				

DAY 1 – Date_____

🕘	**MEAL TRACKING**

SYMPTOM LOG

	🙂	😐	🙁
Previous Night's Sleep			
Bloating			
Gas			
Heartburn			
Constipation			
Acid Reflux			

Number of Eliminations_____

DAY 2 – Date_____

⏰	**MEAL TRACKING**

SYMPTOM LOG

	🙂	😐	☹️
Previous Night's Sleep			
Bloating			
Gas			
Heartburn			
Constipation			
Acid Reflux			

Number of Eliminations_____

DAY 3 – Date_____

🕐	MEAL TRACKING

SYMPTOM LOG

	🙂	😐	🙁
Previous Night's Sleep			
Bloating			
Gas			
Heartburn			
Constipation			
Acid Reflux			

Number of Eliminations_____

DAY 4 – Date_____

🕐	MEAL TRACKING

SYMPTOM LOG

	🙂	😐	🙁
Previous Night's Sleep			
Bloating			
Gas			
Heartburn			
Constipation			
Acid Reflux			

Number of Eliminations_____

DAY 5 – Date_____

🕐	**MEAL TRACKING**

SYMPTOM LOG

	🙂	😐	🙁
Previous Night's Sleep			
Bloating			
Gas			
Heartburn			
Constipation			
Acid Reflux			

Number of Eliminations_____

DAY 6 – Date_____

⏰	**MEAL TRACKING**

SYMPTOM LOG

	🙂	😐	☹️
Previous Night's Sleep			
Bloating			
Gas			
Heartburn			
Constipation			
Acid Reflux			

Number of Eliminations_____

DAY 7 – Date_____

⏰	MEAL TRACKING

SYMPTOM LOG

	🙂	😐	🙁
Previous Night's Sleep			
Bloating			
Gas			
Heartburn			
Constipation			
Acid Reflux			

Number of Eliminations_____

WEEKLY MEAL PLANNER
Week of _____

	BREAKFAST	LUNCH	DINNER	SNACKS
MON				
TUE				
WED				
THU				
FRI				
SAT				
SUN				

DAY 8 – Date_____

🕐	MEAL TRACKING

SYMPTOM LOG

	🙂	😐	🙁
Previous Night's Sleep			
Bloating			
Gas			
Heartburn			
Constipation			
Acid Reflux			

Number of Eliminations_____

DAY 9 – Date_____

🕐	**MEAL TRACKING**

SYMPTOM LOG

	🙂	😐	🙁
Previous Night's Sleep			
Bloating			
Gas			
Heartburn			
Constipation			
Acid Reflux			

Number of Eliminations_____

DAY 10 – Date_____

🕒	**MEAL TRACKING**

SYMPTOM LOG

	🙂	😐	🙁
Previous Night's Sleep			
Bloating			
Gas			
Heartburn			
Constipation			
Acid Reflux			

Number of Eliminations_____

DAY 11 – Date_____

⏲	MEAL TRACKING

SYMPTOM LOG

	🙂	😐	🙁
Previous Night's Sleep			
Bloating			
Gas			
Heartburn			
Constipation			
Acid Reflux			

Number of Eliminations_____

DAY 12 – Date_____

⏰	MEAL TRACKING

SYMPTOM LOG

	🙂	😐	🙁
Previous Night's Sleep			
Bloating			
Gas			
Heartburn			
Constipation			
Acid Reflux			

Number of Eliminations_____

DAY 13 – Date_____

🕐	MEAL TRACKING

SYMPTOM LOG

	🙂	😐	🙁
Previous Night's Sleep			
Bloating			
Gas			
Heartburn			
Constipation			
Acid Reflux			

Number of Eliminations_____

DAY 14 – Date_____

🕐	**MEAL TRACKING**

SYMPTOM LOG

	🙂	😐	🙁
Previous Night's Sleep			
Bloating			
Gas			
Heartburn			
Constipation			
Acid Reflux			

Number of Eliminations_____

WEEKLY MEAL PLANNER
Week of _____

	BREAKFAST	LUNCH	DINNER	SNACKS
MON				
TUE				
WED				
THU				
FRI				
SAT				
SUN				

DAY 15 – Date_____

🕐	MEAL TRACKING

SYMPTOM LOG

	🙂	😐	🙁
Previous Night's Sleep			
Bloating			
Gas			
Heartburn			
Constipation			
Acid Reflux			

Number of Eliminations_____

DAY 16 – Date_____

⏰	MEAL TRACKING

SYMPTOM LOG

	🙂	😐	🙁
Previous Night's Sleep			
Bloating			
Gas			
Heartburn			
Constipation			
Acid Reflux			

Number of Eliminations_____

DAY 17 – Date_____

🕐	**MEAL TRACKING**

SYMPTOM LOG

	🙂	😐	🙁
Previous Night's Sleep			
Bloating			
Gas			
Heartburn			
Constipation			
Acid Reflux			

Number of Eliminations_____

DAY 18 – Date_____

⏰	**MEAL TRACKING**

SYMPTOM LOG

	🙂	😐	🙁
Previous Night's Sleep			
Bloating			
Gas			
Heartburn			
Constipation			
Acid Reflux			

Number of Eliminations_____

DAY 19 – Date_____

🕐	**MEAL TRACKING**

SYMPTOM LOG

	🙂	😐	🙁
Previous Night's Sleep			
Bloating			
Gas			
Heartburn			
Constipation			
Acid Reflux			

Number of Eliminations_____

DAY 20 – Date_____

🕐	**MEAL TRACKING**

SYMPTOM LOG

	🙂	😐	🙁
Previous Night's Sleep			
Bloating			
Gas			
Heartburn			
Constipation			
Acid Reflux			

Number of Eliminations_____

DAY 21 – Date_____

🕐	**MEAL TRACKING**

SYMPTOM LOG

	🙂	😐	🙁
Previous Night's Sleep			
Bloating			
Gas			
Heartburn			
Constipation			
Acid Reflux			

Number of Eliminations_____

WEEKLY MEAL PLANNER
Week of _____

	BREAKFAST	LUNCH	DINNER	SNACKS
MON				
TUE				
WED				
THU				
FRI				
SAT				
SUN				

DAY 22 – Date_____

🕐	MEAL TRACKING

SYMPTOM LOG

	🙂	😐	🙁
Previous Night's Sleep			
Bloating			
Gas			
Heartburn			
Constipation			
Acid Reflux			

Number of Eliminations_____

DAY 23 – Date_____

⏱	**MEAL TRACKING**

SYMPTOM LOG

	🙂	😐	☹
Previous Night's Sleep			
Bloating			
Gas			
Heartburn			
Constipation			
Acid Reflux			

Number of Eliminations_____

DAY 24 – Date_____

⏰	MEAL TRACKING

SYMPTOM LOG

	🙂	😐	🙁
Previous Night's Sleep			
Bloating			
Gas			
Heartburn			
Constipation			
Acid Reflux			

Number of Eliminations_____

DAY 25 – Date_____

🕐	MEAL TRACKING

SYMPTOM LOG

	🙂	😐	🙁
Previous Night's Sleep			
Bloating			
Gas			
Heartburn			
Constipation			
Acid Reflux			

Number of Eliminations_____

DAY 26 – Date_____

⏰	**MEAL TRACKING**

SYMPTOM LOG

	🙂	😐	🙁
Previous Night's Sleep			
Bloating			
Gas			
Heartburn			
Constipation			
Acid Reflux			

Number of Eliminations_____

DAY 27 – Date_____

⏰	**MEAL TRACKING**

SYMPTOM LOG

	🙂	😐	☹️
Previous Night's Sleep			
Bloating			
Gas			
Heartburn			
Constipation			
Acid Reflux			

Number of Eliminations_____

DAY 28 – Date_____

🕒	**MEAL TRACKING**

SYMPTOM LOG

	🙂	😐	🙁
Previous Night's Sleep			
Bloating			
Gas			
Heartburn			
Constipation			
Acid Reflux			

Number of Eliminations_____

WEEKLY MEAL PLANNER
Week of _____

	BREAKFAST	LUNCH	DINNER	SNACKS
MON				
TUE				
WED				
THU				
FRI				
SAT				
SUN				

DAY 29 – Date_____

🕐	MEAL TRACKING

SYMPTOM LOG

	🙂	😐	🙁
Previous Night's Sleep			
Bloating			
Gas			
Heartburn			
Constipation			
Acid Reflux			

Number of Eliminations_____

DAY 30 – Date_____

🕐	**MEAL TRACKING**

SYMPTOM LOG

	🙂	😐	🙁
Previous Night's Sleep			
Bloating			
Gas			
Heartburn			
Constipation			
Acid Reflux			

Number of Eliminations_____

MIDWAY PICTURE

MY WEIGHT_____

WHAT I'M THINKING/HOW I FEEL: _____

_____

_____

_____

_____

_____

_____

DAY 31 – Date_____

ⓛ	MEAL TRACKING

SYMPTOM LOG

	🙂	😐	🙁
Previous Night's Sleep			
Bloating			
Gas			
Heartburn			
Constipation			
Acid Reflux			

Number of Eliminations_____

DAY 32 – Date_____

⏱	MEAL TRACKING

SYMPTOM LOG

	🙂	😐	🙁
Previous Night's Sleep			
Bloating			
Gas			
Heartburn			
Constipation			
Acid Reflux			

Number of Eliminations_____

DAY 33 – Date_____

🕐	**MEAL TRACKING**

SYMPTOM LOG

	🙂	😐	🙁
Previous Night's Sleep			
Bloating			
Gas			
Heartburn			
Constipation			
Acid Reflux			

Number of Eliminations_____

DAY 34 – Date_____

🕐	**MEAL TRACKING**

SYMPTOM LOG

	🙂	😐	🙁
Previous Night's Sleep			
Bloating			
Gas			
Heartburn			
Constipation			
Acid Reflux			

Number of Eliminations_____

DAY 35 – Date_____

🕐	MEAL TRACKING

SYMPTOM LOG

	🙂	😐	🙁
Previous Night's Sleep			
Bloating			
Gas			
Heartburn			
Constipation			
Acid Reflux			

Number of Eliminations_____

WEEKLY MEAL PLANNER
Week of _____

	BREAKFAST	LUNCH	DINNER	SNACKS
MON				
TUE				
WED				
THU				
FRI				
SAT				
SUN				

DAY 36 – Date_____

🕐	MEAL TRACKING

SYMPTOM LOG

	🙂	😐	🙁
Previous Night's Sleep			
Bloating			
Gas			
Heartburn			
Constipation			
Acid Reflux			

Number of Eliminations_____

DAY 37 – Date_____

⏰	MEAL TRACKING

SYMPTOM LOG

	🙂	😐	☹️
Previous Night's Sleep			
Bloating			
Gas			
Heartburn			
Constipation			
Acid Reflux			

Number of Eliminations_____

DAY 38 – Date_____

🕒	**MEAL TRACKING**

SYMPTOM LOG

	🙂	😐	🙁
Previous Night's Sleep			
Bloating			
Gas			
Heartburn			
Constipation			
Acid Reflux			

Number of Eliminations_____

DAY 39 – Date_____

🕐	MEAL TRACKING

SYMPTOM LOG

	🙂	😐	🙁
Previous Night's Sleep			
Bloating			
Gas			
Heartburn			
Constipation			
Acid Reflux			

Number of Eliminations_____

DAY 40 – Date_____

🕐	**MEAL TRACKING**

SYMPTOM LOG

	🙂	😐	🙁
Previous Night's Sleep			
Bloating			
Gas			
Heartburn			
Constipation			
Acid Reflux			

Number of Eliminations_____

DAY 41 – Date_____

⏰	**MEAL TRACKING**

SYMPTOM LOG

	🙂	😐	🙁
Previous Night's Sleep			
Bloating			
Gas			
Heartburn			
Constipation			
Acid Reflux			

Number of Eliminations_____

DAY 42 – Date_____

🕐	**MEAL TRACKING**

SYMPTOM LOG

	🙂	😐	🙁
Previous Night's Sleep			
Bloating			
Gas			
Heartburn			
Constipation			
Acid Reflux			

Number of Eliminations_____

WEEKLY MEAL PLANNER
Week of _____

	BREAKFAST	LUNCH	DINNER	SNACKS
MON				
TUE				
WED				
THU				
FRI				
SAT				
SUN				

DAY 43 – Date_____

🕐	**MEAL TRACKING**

SYMPTOM LOG

	🙂	😐	🙁
Previous Night's Sleep			
Bloating			
Gas			
Heartburn			
Constipation			
Acid Reflux			

Number of Eliminations_____

DAY 44 – Date_____

🕐	MEAL TRACKING

SYMPTOM LOG

	🙂	😐	🙁
Previous Night's Sleep			
Bloating			
Gas			
Heartburn			
Constipation			
Acid Reflux			

Number of Eliminations_____

DAY 45 – Date_____

⏰	**MEAL TRACKING**

SYMPTOM LOG

	🙂	😐	🙁
Previous Night's Sleep			
Bloating			
Gas			
Heartburn			
Constipation			
Acid Reflux			

Number of Eliminations_____

DAY 46 – Date_____

⏰	**MEAL TRACKING**

SYMPTOM LOG

	🙂	😐	🙁
Previous Night's Sleep			
Bloating			
Gas			
Heartburn			
Constipation			
Acid Reflux			

Number of Eliminations_____

DAY 47 – Date_____

🕐	**MEAL TRACKING**

SYMPTOM LOG

	🙂	😐	🙁
Previous Night's Sleep			
Bloating			
Gas			
Heartburn			
Constipation			
Acid Reflux			

Number of Eliminations_____

DAY 48 – Date_____

🕐	MEAL TRACKING

SYMPTOM LOG

	🙂	😐	🙁
Previous Night's Sleep			
Bloating			
Gas			
Heartburn			
Constipation			
Acid Reflux			

Number of Eliminations_____

DAY 49 – Date_____

🕐	**MEAL TRACKING**

SYMPTOM LOG

	🙂	😐	🙁
Previous Night's Sleep			
Bloating			
Gas			
Heartburn			
Constipation			
Acid Reflux			

Number of Eliminations_____

WEEKLY MEAL PLANNER
Week of _____

	BREAKFAST	LUNCH	DINNER	SNACKS
MON				
TUE				
WED				
THU				
FRI				
SAT				
SUN				

DAY 50 – Date_____

🕐	**MEAL TRACKING**

SYMPTOM LOG

	🙂	😐	🙁
Previous Night's Sleep			
Bloating			
Gas			
Heartburn			
Constipation			
Acid Reflux			

Number of Eliminations_____

DAY 51 – Date_____

⏰	MEAL TRACKING

SYMPTOM LOG

	🙂	😐	🙁
Previous Night's Sleep			
Bloating			
Gas			
Heartburn			
Constipation			
Acid Reflux			

Number of Eliminations_____

DAY 52 – Date_____

🕐	**MEAL TRACKING**

SYMPTOM LOG

	🙂	😐	🙁
Previous Night's Sleep			
Bloating			
Gas			
Heartburn			
Constipation			
Acid Reflux			

Number of Eliminations_____

DAY 53 – Date_____

⏰	MEAL TRACKING

SYMPTOM LOG

	🙂	😐	🙁
Previous Night's Sleep			
Bloating			
Gas			
Heartburn			
Constipation			
Acid Reflux			

Number of Eliminations_____

DAY 54 – Date_____

🕐	MEAL TRACKING

SYMPTOM LOG

	🙂	😐	🙁
Previous Night's Sleep			
Bloating			
Gas			
Heartburn			
Constipation			
Acid Reflux			

Number of Eliminations_____

DAY 55 – Date_____

🕐	**MEAL TRACKING**

SYMPTOM LOG

	🙂	😐	🙁
Previous Night's Sleep			
Bloating			
Gas			
Heartburn			
Constipation			
Acid Reflux			

Number of Eliminations_____

DAY 56 – Date_____

🕐	**MEAL TRACKING**

SYMPTOM LOG

	🙂	😐	🙁
Previous Night's Sleep			
Bloating			
Gas			
Heartburn			
Constipation			
Acid Reflux			

Number of Eliminations_____

WEEKLY MEAL PLANNER
Week of _____

	BREAKFAST	LUNCH	DINNER	SNACKS
MON				
TUE				
WED				
THU				
FRI				
SAT				
SUN				

DAY 57 – Date_____

🕐	MEAL TRACKING

SYMPTOM LOG

	🙂	😐	🙁
Previous Night's Sleep			
Bloating			
Gas			
Heartburn			
Constipation			
Acid Reflux			

Number of Eliminations_____

DAY 58 – Date_____

⏰	**MEAL TRACKING**

SYMPTOM LOG

	🙂	😐	🙁
Previous Night's Sleep			
Bloating			
Gas			
Heartburn			
Constipation			
Acid Reflux			

Number of Eliminations_____

DAY 59 – Date_____

⏰	**MEAL TRACKING**

SYMPTOM LOG

	🙂	😐	🙁
Previous Night's Sleep			
Bloating			
Gas			
Heartburn			
Constipation			
Acid Reflux			

Number of Eliminations_____

DAY 60 – Date_____

⏰	**MEAL TRACKING**

SYMPTOM LOG

	🙂	😐	🙁
Previous Night's Sleep			
Bloating			
Gas			
Heartburn			
Constipation			
Acid Reflux			

Number of Eliminations_____

AFTER PICTURE

MY WEIGHT_____

WHAT I'M THINKING/HOW I FEEL: _____

_____

_____

_____

_____

_____

_____

FAVORITE RECIPES

Recipe Name: _____
*Serves:*_____

Oven Temp_____Prep Time_____Cook Time _____

Ingredients:

Preparation Directions:

Cooking Directions:

Notes:

FAVORITE RECIPES

Recipe Name: _____
*Serves:*_____

Oven Temp_____Prep Time_____Cook Time _____

Ingredients:

_____   _____

_____   _____

_____   _____

_____   _____

Preparation Directions:

_____
_____
_____
_____
_____

Cooking Directions:

_____
_____
_____
_____
_____

Notes:

_____
_____
_____
_____
_____

FAVORITE RECIPES

Recipe Name: _____
*Serves:*_____

Oven Temp_____Prep Time_____Cook Time _____

Ingredients:

_____   _____

_____   _____

_____   _____

_____   _____

Preparation Directions:
_____
_____
_____
_____
_____

Cooking Directions:
_____
_____
_____
_____
_____

Notes:
_____
_____
_____
_____
_____

FAVORITE RECIPES

Recipe Name: _____
*Serves:*_____

Oven Temp_____Prep Time_____Cook Time _____

Ingredients:

_____   _____

_____   _____

_____   _____

_____   _____

Preparation Directions:

_____
_____
_____
_____
_____

Cooking Directions:

_____
_____
_____
_____
_____

Notes:

_____
_____
_____
_____
_____

FAVORITE RECIPES

Recipe Name: _____
*Serves:*_____

Oven Temp_____Prep Time_____Cook Time _____

Ingredients:

_____   _____

_____   _____

_____   _____

_____   _____

Preparation Directions:

_____
_____
_____
_____
_____

Cooking Directions:

_____
_____
_____
_____
_____

Notes:

_____
_____
_____
_____
_____

FAVORITE RECIPES

Recipe Name: _____
*Serves:*_____

Oven Temp_____Prep Time_____Cook Time _____

Ingredients:

_____   _____

_____   _____

_____   _____

_____   _____

Preparation Directions:

_____
_____
_____
_____
_____

Cooking Directions:

_____
_____
_____
_____
_____

Notes:

_____
_____
_____
_____
_____

# FAVORITE RECIPES

Recipe Name: _____
*Serves:*_____

Oven Temp_____Prep Time_____Cook Time _____

Ingredients:

_____   _____

_____   _____

_____   _____

_____   _____

Preparation Directions:

_____
_____
_____
_____
_____

Cooking Directions:

_____
_____
_____
_____
_____

Notes:

_____
_____
_____
_____
_____

FAVORITE RECIPES

Recipe Name: _____
*Serves:*_____

Oven Temp_____Prep Time_____Cook Time _____

Ingredients:

_____   _____

_____   _____

_____   _____

_____   _____

Preparation Directions:

_____
_____
_____
_____
_____

Cooking Directions:

_____
_____
_____
_____
_____

Notes:

_____
_____
_____
_____
_____

NOTES

NOTES

NOTES

NOTES

SHOPPING LIST

SHOPPING LIST

SHOPPING LIST

CPSIA information can be obtained at www.ICGtesting.com
Printed in the USA
BVOW04s1842190115

383981BV00014B/394/P